D0442909

Hillsboro Public Library
Hillsboro, OR
A member of Washington County
COOPERATIVE LIBRARY SERVICES

WHOLE BEAUTY

Essential Oils

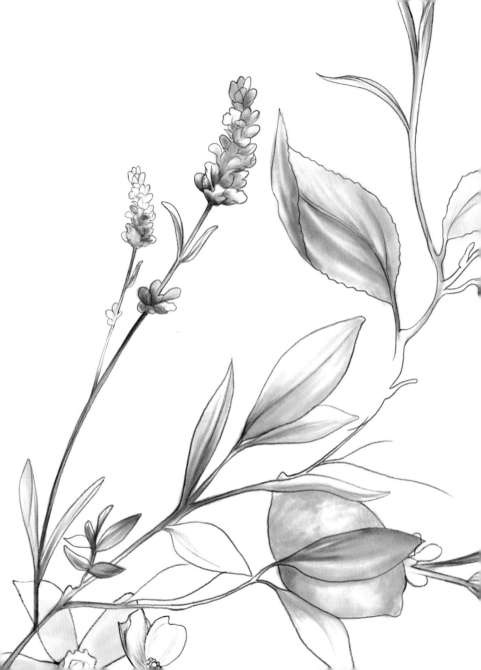

WHOLE BEAUTY

Essential Oils

Homemade Recipes for
Clean Beauty and Household Care

SHIVA ROSE

ARTISAN I NEW YORK

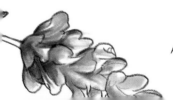

CONTENTS

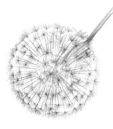

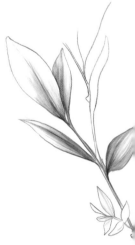

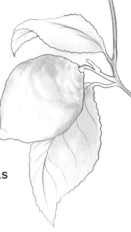

Introduction:
Essential Oils

Essential oils are a gift from the natural world.
The name comes from the term *quintessential
oils*, which is based on the idea that the fifth
element (after fire, earth, air, and water) was
ether, or "quintessence." People believed that
these oils actually captured the spirit of the plant.
Essential oils can be made from bark, leaves, petals,
stems, and roots through processes like steam
distillation, cold-pressing, and resin tapping (it
all depends on the individual plant). As they are
highly concentrated, a little goes a long way.

Essential oils have been used in healing for thousands
of years, in cultures from Greek to Persian, Roman
to Assyrian, and essential oil vessels have even been
found in Egyptian tombs. Ancient priestesses would
carry different resins or essential oils in pouches
against their bodies for power and protection.
Essential oils offer speedy remedies that help us
to heal just by removing a cap and breathing in.
Different essential oils can help to improve mood,
lower stress, reduce pain, quell nausea, banish
headaches, balance hormones, induce sleep, heal
cuts, and soothe insect bites. Used as household

cleaners, they will help to rid your home of toxic chemicals. When you apply essential oils to the skin (dilute them with jojoba oil first, if they are not already diluted; check the label), they are absorbed into the bloodstream, and through inhalation, they go directly to the brain, which is why it is so important to use organic oils from reputable producers (I list a few of my favorites in the Resources section).

Essential oils can play a big role in your beauty and wellness practices and enliven your rituals with healing and fragrance. They are lovely when applied to the temples, the soles of the feet, pulse points, or pressure points. Essential oils can be used throughout the day: In the morning, try energizing and uplifting oils like peppermint and lemon; oils that help you focus and revive you, like frankincense and sandalwood, can help get you through a busy afternoon; and soothing, relaxing oils like lavender are good to use before going to bed or when you are traveling.

To inhale them, put a few drops on a cotton ball or a tissue, hold it to your face, and breathe in deeply. Use them in an essential oil diffuser to scent a room, or put a few drops in the linen closet.

Be sure to test your sensitivity to an essential oil by first applying a drop to the inside of your arm.

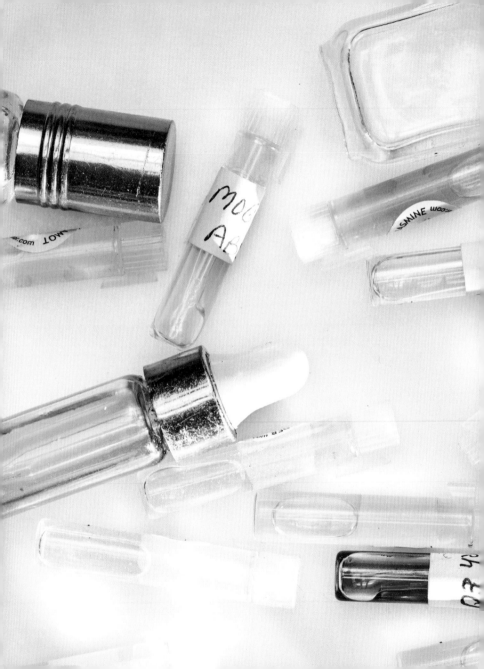

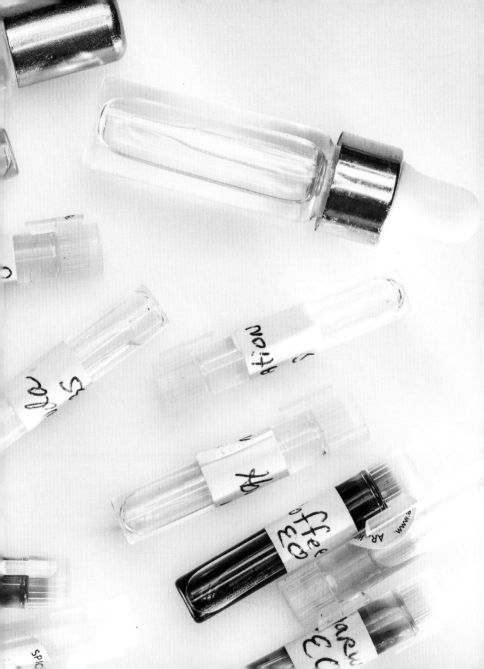

ESSENTIAL ESSENTIAL OILS

Following are the oils I like to have on hand.

FRANKINCENSE OIL

This ancient oil promotes an overall sense of well-being. It helps to relieve inflammation, boosts your immune system, aids in digestion after a heavy meal, and relieves and eases premenstrual symptoms and cramps. Its astringent properties help kill germs on the skin, and it has even been shown to fight some cancer cells.

LAVENDER OIL

Lavender oil is a go-to classic, but you can also choose a different flower oil, such as geranium, clary sage, rose, neroli, or jasmine. These oils will soothe your nerves and help you relax, and you can add drops to your skin and body oils, or anoint pulse points, to increase feelings of sensuality and attractiveness. Flower oils can help lift your mood and transition you back to your emotional and creative self after too many long hours at work. They also can be used to make closets and nurseries smell light and lovely.

LEMON OIL

Lemon oil is an instant mood booster. Massaging a few drops into the soles of your feet can help wake you up when you're feeling sluggish. Lemon helps decongest the liver, balance blood sugar, and ease hunger. For people used to being in the spotlight, lemon helps them to find gratifying pathways and peace of mind without external validation, as it clears the auric fields and resets your olfactory senses. It is a great oil to take on vacation.

PEPPERMINT OIL

Peppermint oil delivers an icy blast on a hot day. Cooling and soothing, it helps alleviate muscle pain and can calm an upset stomach or a throbbing head. Breathing it in or massaging it into the chest can help with respiratory issues from colds or allergies. This is an oil that stimulates creativity.

ROSEMARY OIL

Rosemary oil relieves stress and anxiety while boosting clarity and focus. It is a great aid when studying for a test or preparing for a big event that will require lots of concentration and planning. It promotes physical stamina and emotional strength. When massaged into the scalp, it promotes hair growth and prevents dandruff, and it also helps increase circulation, which makes it a wonderful addition to massage and body oils.

SANDALWOOD OIL

If you can afford some high-quality sandalwood oil, it is a sensual and luxurious addition to your essential oil regimen. It helps to relax breathing and serves as an antidepressant. It increases vitality and is a superior oil for meditation, as it helps you center yourself and connect with the source of all being.

TEA TREE OIL

Tea tree oil is a wonderful alternative to antifungal products. It is a powerful antiseptic that can be used to treat acne, bacterial infections, insect bites, dandruff, and fungal infections like candida, nail fungus, and ringworm. *Note: While many essential oils (like oregano or cinnamon) can be taken internally, never ingest tea tree oil.*

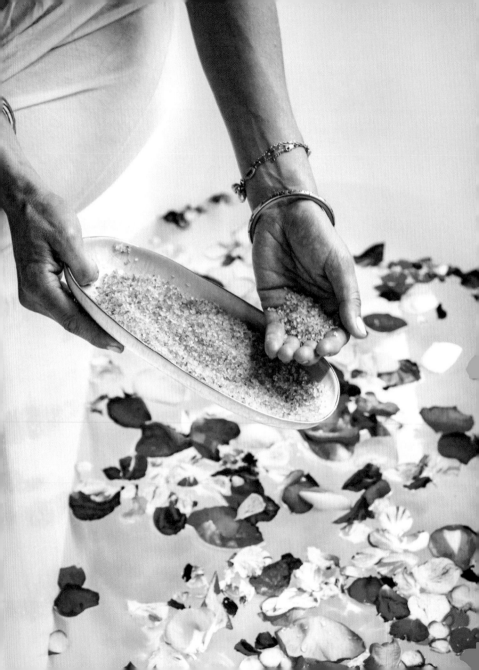

Healing Baths

In ancient times, bathing was regarded as a gift of health from the gods themselves. Making baths a ritual can be a therapeutic activity. Taking a bath is the perfect way to have nourishing alone time and create a bit of sanctuary for yourself. Baths are cleansing and can enhance physical and mental energy, remove negativity, and relax your body and mind. They're also a wonderful way to soak up the deeply therapeutic medicine of essential oils and other good-for-the-skin ingredients (see Resources for suggestions on where to shop). I like to add crystals to baths for clearing, balancing, and healing (see page 21).

Cleopatra's Secret
Bath Recipe

This is an incredibly nourishing treat for the skin. The lactic acid in the milk (I prefer raw, as it has more enzymes and is cleaner) works to remove impurities. The honey is like food for the skin, and rose opens the heart and is anti-aging. After this bath, your skin will be smooth, soft, and opulently scented. It is also ideal for balancing the Pitta and Vata doshas (see page 77).

3 cups cow's or goat's milk, preferably raw

1 tablespoon raw honey

10 drops of rose essential oil

A handful of organic fresh or dried rose petals

Fill the tub with water that is the ideal temperature for you. Add the milk, honey, essential oil, and rose petals before you step in. Soak for 20 minutes or more.

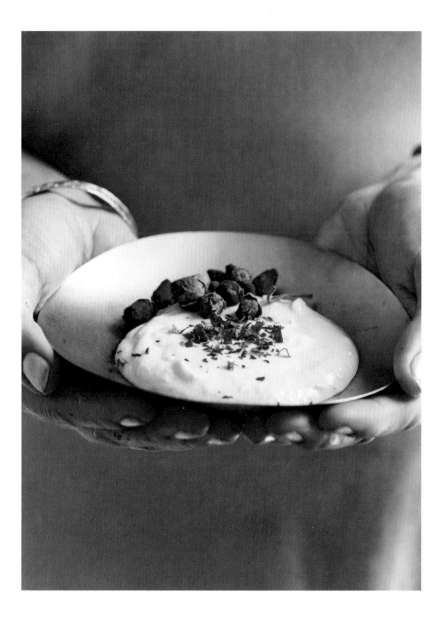

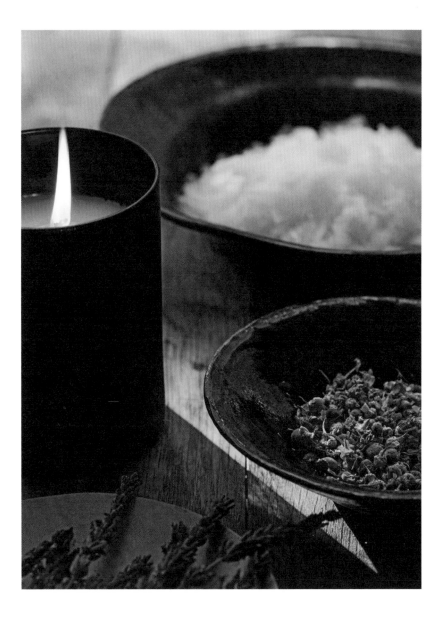

Relaxing Mineral Bath

One of my favorite relaxing baths for all doshas
(see page 77) is a magnesium bath. Most of
us are lacking magnesium due to depleted
foods that are the result of overtaxed soil
beds. Magnesium is essential for healthy
skin and hair, aids sleep, and can promote a
profound sense of calm and well-being.

1 cup magnesium flakes

10 drops of a relaxing essential oil (I like
   chamomile or lavender)

Fill the tub with water that is the ideal temperature
for you. Add the magnesium flakes and essential oil
before you step in. Soak for 20 minutes or more.

Awakening Bath

Ginger is an excellent tonic for waking up the senses, and this bath revives and relaxes you before a night out. Or if you are sick with a fever, a ginger bath can help you sweat out toxins and soothe sore muscles. It is also good for balancing Kapha dominance (see page 77).

½ cup freshly grated ginger, or 1 teaspoon
    powdered ginger
1 teaspoon almond oil
10 drops of neroli essential oil

Fill the tub with water that is the ideal temperature for you. Add the ginger, almond oil, and essential oil before you step in. Soak for 20 minutes or more.

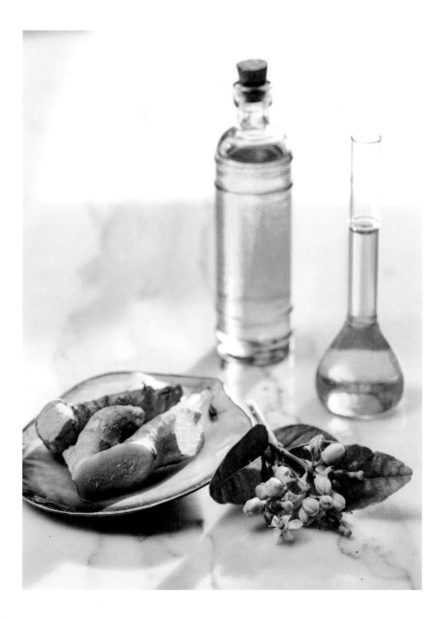

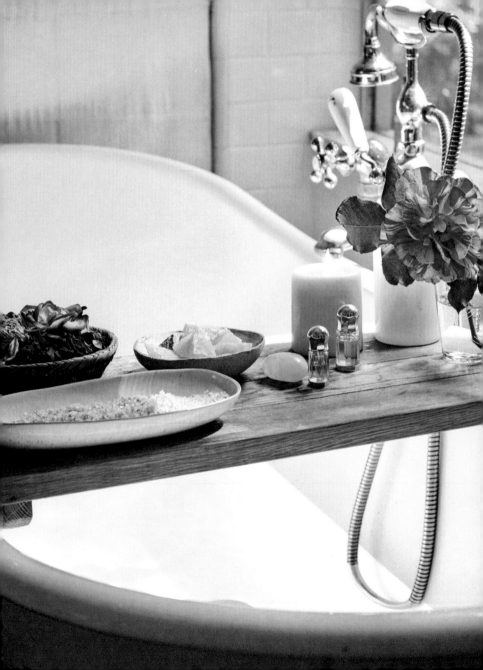

Clearing Baths

Deborah Hanekamp, a friend and healer, introduced me to the idea of using crystals in a bath, and I have been doing it ever since. When combined with salt, herbs, and flowers in the bath, the crystals' energy is amplified. The use of crystals also makes for a visually beautiful treatment.

To Bring in Love

A handful of pink Himalayan salt

A handful of rose petals

A handful of dried lavender

Rose quartz crystals

10 drops of rose or lavender essential oil

To Cleanse Negative Energy

A handful of sea salt

A handful of white sage

A handful of rosemary

Black tourmaline crystals

10 drops of rosemary or sage essential oil

Fill the tub with water that is the ideal temperature for you. Add the ingredients of your choosing before you step in. Soak for 20 minutes or more.

My Favorite Crystals

Aside from just their sheer beauty, crystals help us bring the desired energy and vibrations into our lives. Shopping for crystals is like falling in love. You are drawn to certain ones for specific reasons, so go with your gut and don't overthink it! It's important to note that the color varies from crystal to crystal, and just because you might come across one that does not match its typical color, it doesn't mean that it's less powerful. Here are some of my favorites.

Amethyst

A lovely lavender, amethyst helps to heal the heart and soothe the nervous system. It is the stone of spirituality and contentment, and it promotes calm.

Black Tourmaline

Dark and shiny, black tourmaline releases negative energy, provides protection, and shields from harmful EMF (electromagnetic field) rays. I keep a large piece of black tourmaline by my computer.

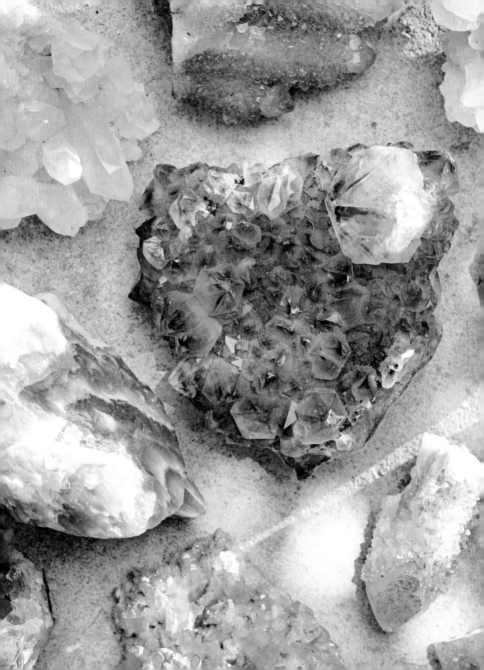

Citrine

A honey-yellow hue, citrine promotes abundance and financial stability. A stone of manifestation, it can help bring your desires into being.

Jade

A delicate mint green, jade balances energy and can help bring in prosperity. It calms the mind and enhances our life force. Jade has been said to bless whatever it touches.

Labradorite

A range of different, subtle colors, labradorite inspires intuition and aids in connecting to higher realms and overcoming emotional blocks.

Moonstone

Shimmery like a pearl, moonstone connects us to the feminine by representing the power of the moon. It can also help to enhance our intuition, balance the chakras (see page 83), and promote a sense of calm.

Morganite

A pale peachy-pink stone, morganite is a mysterious crystal. It helps to heal and release old wounds and traumas, and it is used to bring in your soul mate.

Rose Quartz

A lovely light pink, rose quartz has a soft, feminine energy that inspires beauty. It helps with healing, to open the heart, and to bring love into your life.

Smoky Quartz

A clear gray, smoky quartz helps with organization and clarity. It releases negativity and promotes protection. It is a powerful grounding stone that is often used in meditation and is helpful when praying to ancestors and for anchoring yourself in the natural world.

Tiger's Eye

A beautiful blend of dark and light brown, tiger's eye inspires and aids in decision-making. It releases negativity and provides clarity.

CARING FOR YOUR CRYSTALS

CHARGING

To charge a crystal is to imbue it with energy and intentions. There is no right or wrong way to do this. You can charge your crystals anywhere you think they will absorb positive energy. Bathe them in sunlight or moonlight. (I tend to see sunlight as a more masculine, active energy and moonlight as a more feminine, receptive energy.) Or charge them on your altar (or any place that is sacred to you). Simply place the crystal on the altar, light a candle, and spend a few moments meditating, imagining your intentions and energy going into the crystal.

CLEANSING

Cleansing crystals allows them to release all of the energy that they have absorbed. Always cleanse crystals before their first use, and also after rituals or experiencing tough situations. Charging crystals under the sun or moon also clears them, but once a month, fill a big bowl with water, then add a handful of pink Himalayan salt, place your crystals in the saltwater, and let them sit overnight. In the morning, dispose of the water by throwing it outside, and rinse and dry your crystals.

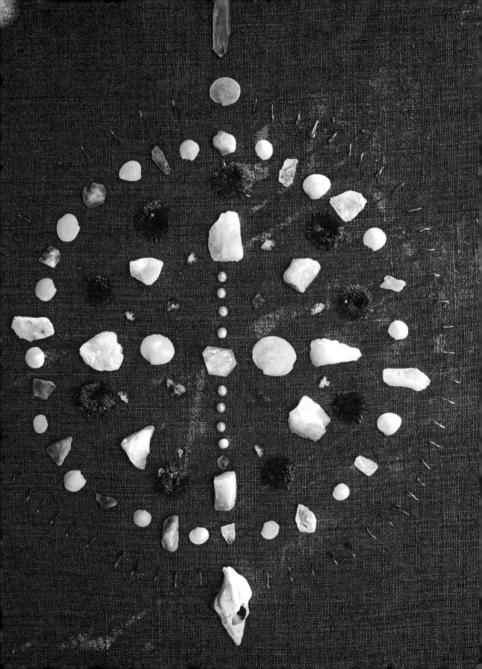

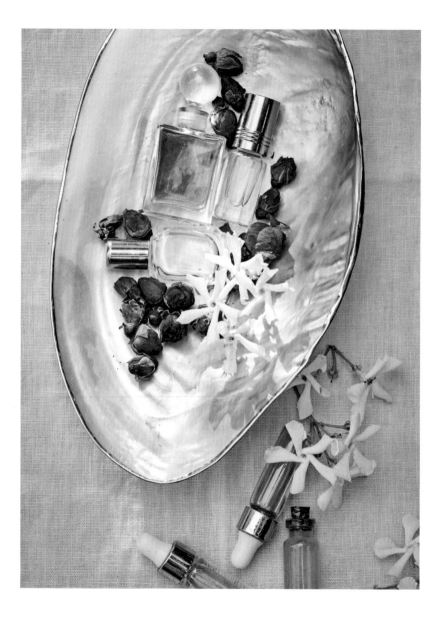

Essential Oils for Daily Use

Essential oils can be of great use to you in lessening your daily exposure to toxic chemicals in personal-care products. We absorb so much more than we are aware of, and to limit and ideally eliminate these hormone-disrupting chemicals is key to leading a life of health and vitality. The recipes that follow smell clean and fresh and are also fun to make.

Hydrosols

No matter what they might claim on the label, many modern moisturizers actually dry out your skin rather than nourish and nurture it. As we age, our skin stops producing as much oil, so we need to take extra care to replenish it, and spritzing throughout the day is a great way to help keep skin hydrated and supple. Hydrosols provide a centering burst of moisture and refreshment wherever you are and whenever you need it. I keep them in the car to bring a little peace when I'm stuck in traffic, and I take them when I travel by plane. I use them regularly to cool down on hot days, and also to clear space for meditation and rituals.

I encourage you to get creative, adapt, and play with these recipes until you've made something that is uniquely perfect for you. Create whatever calls to you in that moment. Adding crystals helps to enhance the desired vibrations and energy.

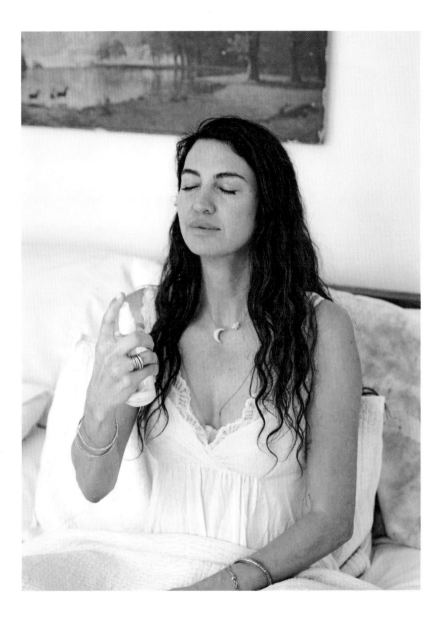

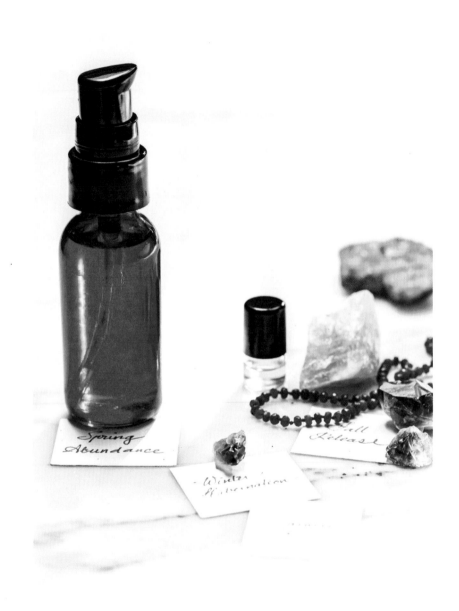

Seasonal Hydrosols

One way to balance your skin during changing weather is to use a specific hydrosol for the corresponding season.

4 ounces purified water

1 drop of colloidal silver to act as a natural preservative (you can buy this at most health food stores)

Essential oils and crystals for the season of your choosing (see the following pages)

Glass spray bottle

Fill the spray bottle with the water and colloidal silver. Add the essential oils of your choosing and shake to mix. A good starting point is five drops of each oil, then you can add more of the individual oils until you've created a scent that is pleasing to you. Add the crystals and spritz as needed. You cannot overuse hydrosols. Stored out of the sun, they should last about a month.

Continued

SPRING ABUNDANCE

Essential Oils

Lily, neroli, rose, sweet orange, sweet pea

Crystals

Amethyst for courage and protection

Rose quartz for love and healing

SUMMER JOY

Essential Oils

Cucumber, gardenia, jasmine, lavender, lemon, lemongrass, mint, rose geranium, rosemary

Crystals

Moonstone for sleep and beauty

Watermelon tourmaline for compassion and balance

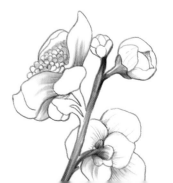

FALL RELEASE

Essential Oils
Amber, oakmoss, patchouli, sage, vanilla

Crystals
Black tourmaline for clearing negativity
Citrine for psychic awareness
Jade for longevity and prosperity

WINTER HIBERNATION

Essential Oils
Cedar, cinnamon, clove, cypress, juniper, patchouli,
pine, sandalwood

Crystals
Garnet for energy and to strengthen your aura
Lemon quartz for clarity and abundance
Pearl for luck and money

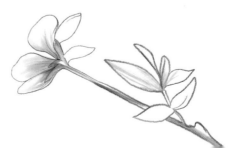

Toners

The microbiome of skin mirrors the microbiome of soil. If you don't have healthy soil, you won't have healthy food. Just the same, if you don't have a healthy microbiome on your face, you won't have healthy skin. The microbiome is made out of good bacteria, so you don't want to strip it from your skin. Toners feed your skin certain nutrient-rich elements, which help to nourish the microbiome, allowing it to flourish. This can ease dry skin and help stop breakouts.

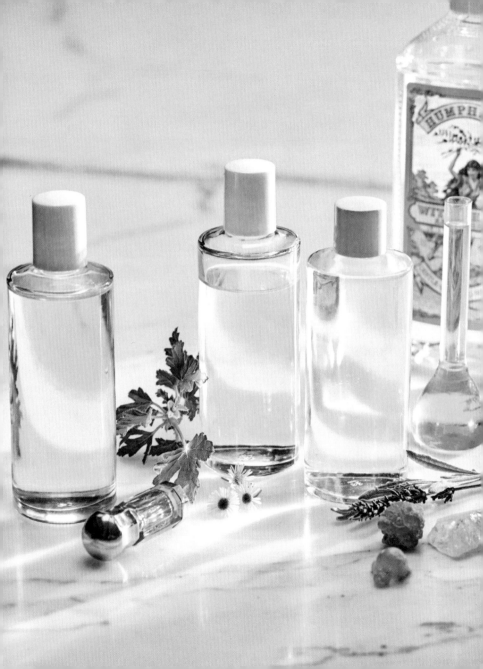

Toner Blends

I apply toner after I cleanse and again after I put on an oil. Toners add minerals to the skin and set the groundwork for moisturizing, and they can also serve in a pinch when you can't do a full cleanse.

6 ounces purified water

1 drop of colloidal silver to act as a natural
    preservative (you can buy this at most
    health food stores)

Ingredients for your skin type

Glass bottle with cap

For Normal / Combination Skin

1 tablespoon witch hazel

5 drops of lavender oil

3 drops of grapefruit oil

3 drops of Virginia cedarwood oil

For Acne-Prone / Oily Skin

1 tablespoon apple cider vinegar

5 drops of lavender oil

5 drops of tea tree oil

3 drops of grapefruit oil

2 drops of lemongrass oil

For Aging / Dry Skin

1 tablespoon aloe vera

10 drops of petitgrain oil

5 drops of frankincense oil

2 drops of geranium oil

2 drops of carrot seed oil (or 3 drops of
Roman chamomile oil, if you don't like
the carrot seed scent)

Put the water, colloidal silver, and ingredients that
pertain to your skin type in the glass bottle. Tightly
close the cap and shake to mix. Apply with a cotton
pad. Store out of direct sunlight for up to 3 months.

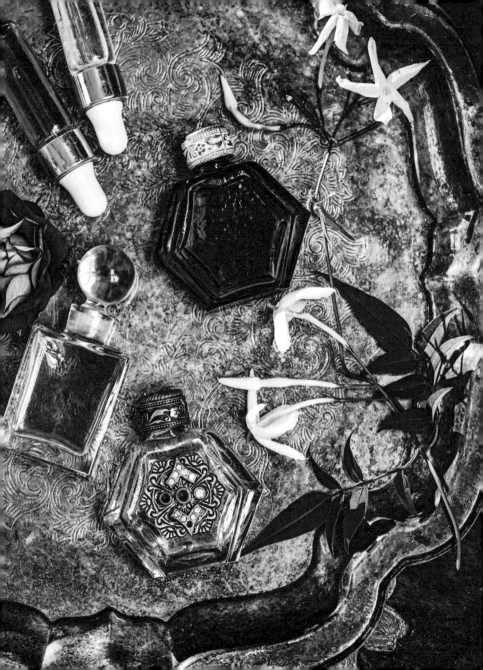

Perfumes

In a time when almost every scent is recognizable, or easily accessible via the internet, why not create a signature scent that evokes where you are in the moment? Just like choosing an outfit depends on your mood, you can do the same thing with hand-blended custom perfumes.

The beautiful thing about blending essential oil perfumes is that there is no right or wrong way to do it. You simply follow your nose until you have something that agrees with you. In this way, it is easy to create a signature scent, or you can combine different oils that you alternate depending on your mood or the occasion.

Goddess Perfumes

I love invoking the goddesses (see page 44) in my rituals, and I frequently set up their images and offerings on my altars. I created these perfume blends as a way to take the goddesses with me wherever I go. If I am standing in line, caught in traffic, or otherwise involved in a stressful situation, all I need to do is dab a little of one of these scents on my wrists to invoke Lalita's love or Artemis's courage. I blend them in front of my altar, on a Friday night to honor Venus, or during a waning moon, when the moon is preparing to renew. After the scent has been mixed, I will leave it on the altar for a few days to charge it with goddess energy.

5 drops of each essential oil for the goddess of your choosing (or adjust to your preference)
1 tablespoon jojoba oil

Glass bottle with stopper or rollerball applicator (common sizes are 10 and 15 milliliters)

Place drops of the essential oils of your choice into the glass bottle or rollerball applicator. Top with the jojoba oil. Add the stopper and shake to mix. Charge the perfume on your altar for a few days before applying. Store out of direct sunlight for up to 3 months.

Venus
Jasmine, rose, ylang-ylang

Freyja
Musk, patchouli, sandalwood

Parvati
Cardamom, vanilla, ylang-ylang

Lakshmi
Lily, rose, sandalwood

Lalita
Amber, musk, vanilla

Artemis
Cedar, frankincense, juniper

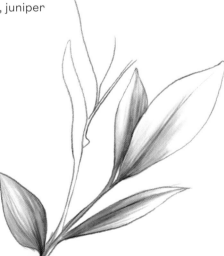

Invoking the Goddesses

I have always called myself a feminine feminist, a phrase Anaïs Nin coined so perfectly. I love using the feminine within me to bring more power and sensuality to women everywhere. Women today live in the masculine energy more than ever, and we are now the providers in so many ways. This can be fulfilling, yet exhausting. Bringing the goddess energy into our lives helps us to balance ourselves and the world around us. The more we become familiar with the goddesses, the more we learn to recognize and acknowledge them.

The goddesses help us to break out of a rut we may be stuck in and celebrate other aspects of who we are, honoring all the dimensions of our lives.

Working with a goddess is developing a personal relationship with her and learning to approach and honor her in a way that feels individual and true to you. On the following pages are examples of how I speak to and call in my favorite goddesses. You do not need to follow these guidelines explicitly, as long as your intention is clear and you are working from a mindful, heartfelt place. Feel free to alter the prayers. The objects are suggestions of what to add

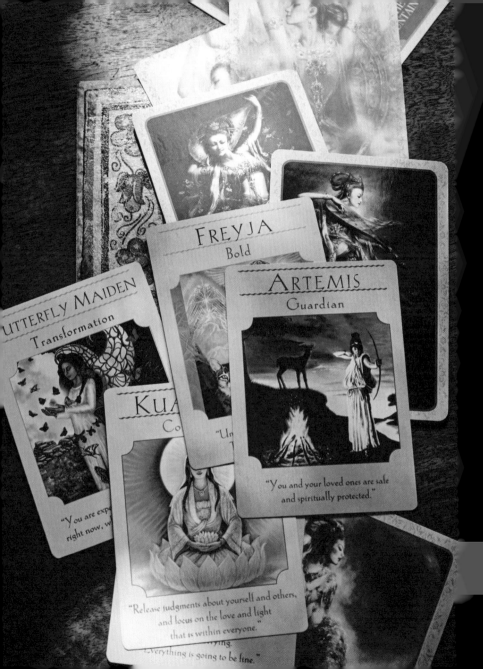

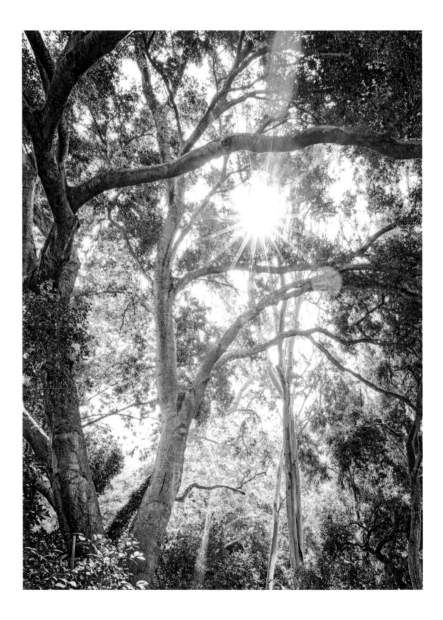

to your altar to call in each particular goddess, but again, you may use whatever is most sacred to you.

A note on chakras as they relate to the goddesses: Chakra means "wheel" in Sanskrit, and the chakras are the seven turning wheels of our energy field (or subtle body). The chakras can be found from the top of the head down to the bottom of the spine. When they are active and spinning, they brighten our aura. When they are closed and stagnant, our aura dims. When our chakras are balanced and working together, we feel confident, calm, and energized, both grounded and in touch with our divine self. For more about chakras, see page 83.

Venus

Venus (or Aphrodite in ancient Greece) is the ancient Roman goddess of love, sex, fertility, abundance, and harvest. When you honor Venus, you are evoking the feminine, the fertile, and the forces of beauty, compassion, and love. You can bring out the Venus in you when you nourish yourself.

Venus came from the sea and was born in water. Every year in ancient Rome, on the first day of April, women lowered the statue of Venus into water and ritually bathed her in honor of feminine sexuality and sensuality. So one way to acknowledge Venus and this ancient ritual is with a bath. Add rose petals and rose essential oil, or go bathe in a lake or the ocean. Venus reminds you to treat yourself the way you want to be treated by others.

A Prayer for Venus

Dear Venus, I am calling upon you to join me here today. I am calling upon your shining starlight to open my crown chakra and breathe love into my heart. I ask for your guidance in bringing me closer to loved ones and healing myself from past wounds. I ask that I use your pink-white energy to bring beauty to all I do. I ask that I can bring healing through my work and a celebration of all that is you.

Sacred Objects for Venus

Red roses, mirrors, rose quartz, luscious fruit, chocolates, milk, honey, images of Venus by the old masters, seashells, pearls—things that bring you joy.

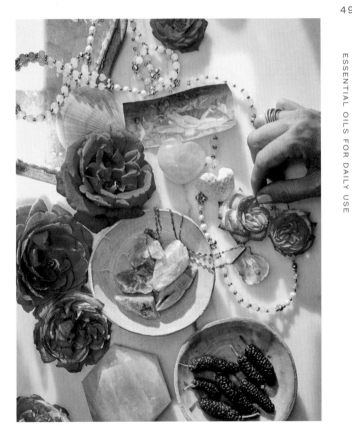

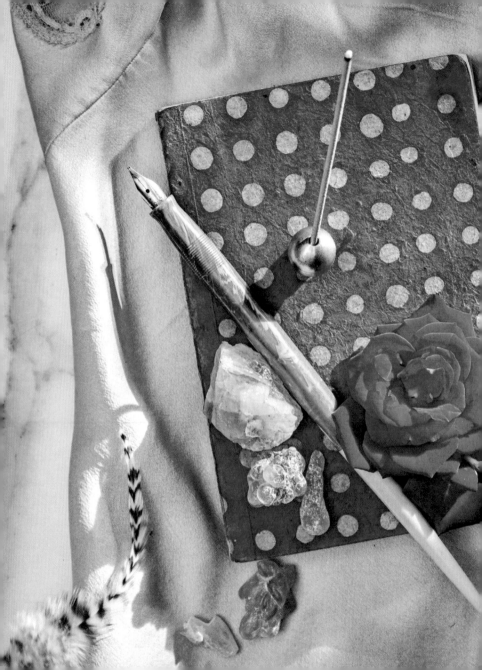

Freyja

Freyja is the Norse goddess of love and fertility. She's one of the most powerful deities and can aid in healing past traumas. She's very sensual and can bring sexuality and wildness into your life. She is seen with wings or wearing feathers and is represented by birds of prey like hawks, falcons, and eagles. She will help you to become more magnetic, own your energy, and ignite fires in your lower chakras.

A Prayer for Freyja

Dear Freyja, please allow me to ignite my sexual identity and my sexual power. Please allow me to heal any past wounds that are keeping me from fulfilling my desires. Allow me to connect to my internal fire and to awaken my lower chakras.

Sacred Objects for Freyja

Take out a pen and write a list of things you wish to attract. Light a candle to symbolize Freyja's flame, and place the list and a piece of beautiful lingerie on your altar. Anoint your altar with musk essential oil. Put on some music that will make you dance with abandon. Go on arduous hikes in the wild and bring home a beautiful rock that symbolizes strength.

Parvati

Parvati is the Hindu goddess of love, seduction, and luminosity. She's a truth seeker, a mother, and wife to Shiva, the god of the yogis. She's very romantic. When she fell in love with Shiva, he wanted nothing to do with her, yet she waited for him until he changed his mind. She never gave up, and in the end, they became a powerful couple who changed the world with their deep love.

Call on Parvati to enhance your relationship, to summon your future love, and to bring protection to your home and family. She embodies kindness, grace, and strength and is a reminder to women that we can be strong and feminine at the same time.

A Prayer for Parvati

Dear Parvati, I call upon your divine energy to bless my home, my family, and my beloved. I call upon your gracious nature to imbue my workspace and all my creations with your honor and blessings. Nurture me so that I may be able to nurture my children and my beloved. Allow me to have your grace, patience, focus, and open and loving heart in all matters of love in my life.

Sacred Objects for Parvati

Think of Parvati as a queen and make your offerings accordingly: jasmine essential oil, fruit, incense, gold, amethyst, crowns, pictures of your children, rubies, aquamarine, hibiscus flowers.

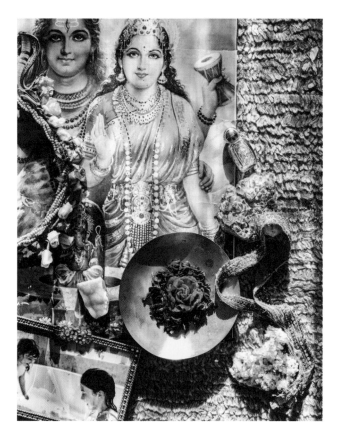

Lakshmi

Lakshmi is the Hindu goddess of fortune and beauty. Like Venus, she came from the sea. When she was born, she emerged fully grown on a pink lotus flower rising up from the water. Lakshmi is a powerful ally to call on to help fulfill professional aspirations, including achieving financial success. She inspires confidence, because confidence leads to abundance. She is a peacemaker and the goddess of working mothers. She's also attracted to cleanliness, so it's good to tidy up your workspace so that she will be drawn in. I generally do a good cleaning on the new moon (for new beginnings). Lakshmi loves music, so another way to honor her is to put some on and sing or dance! *Shanti* means "peace," and "Shanti shanti shanti" is one of her mantras.

A Prayer for Lakshmi

Dear Lakshmi, I call upon you today and ask that you guide me with your wisdom. Allow me to bring more abundance and blessings into my world so that I can help myself and others. Allow me to feel deserving of success and bounty. Allow me to use my good fortune for the betterment of my community and planet.

Sacred Objects for Lakshmi

A beautiful shawl, pink or red flowers, gold coins, lotus flowers, ylang-ylang essential oil, jewelry, fans. Clean your house in her honor and put a picture of her above the stove so that the heat can activate her powers.

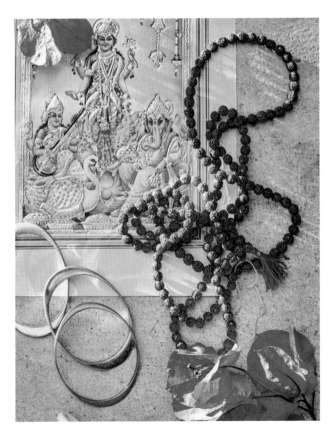

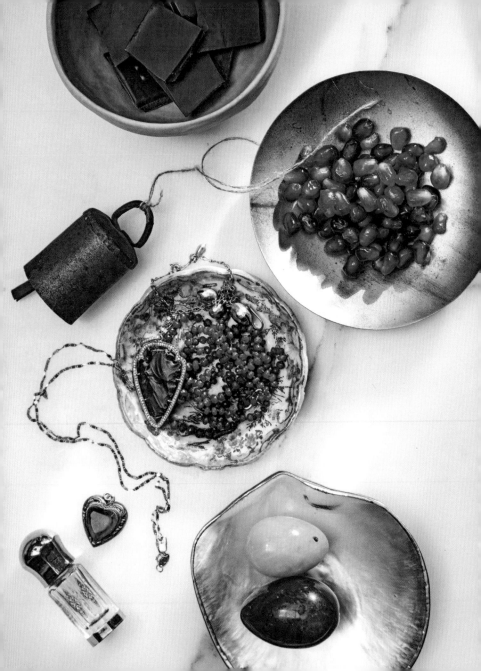

Lalita

Lalita is a yogic goddess who is all about flirtation, sensuality, and childlike fun. She reminds us that life should include lots of laughter and love. Lalita is also known for her beautiful dark hair, so summon her during hair treatments. She brings confidence and a sense of adventure, and she activates the erotic.

A Prayer for Lalita

Dear Lalita, goddess of desire, please magnetize my erotic feminine nature. Please bestow your energy on me and help me activate my sensuality and joy. Send me your wisdom and compassion regarding matters of the heart. Allow me to bring healing through love and my sensual nature.

Sacred Objects for Lalita

Perfume, pomegranates, berries, rubies, bells, arrows, some lubricant or body oil, chocolate, an image of your lover. Or put on some music that creates an atmosphere you feel vibrant in. Do a dance just for yourself, or massage your beloved with a body oil infused with vanilla essential oil in her honor.

Artemis

Artemis (Diana in ancient Rome) is the ancient Greek goddess of the hunt and embodies independence and passion. She can help you advance in your career and pursue new opportunities. She has a laser focus and does not apologize for being self-reliant. I like to think of her as the lady of the wild things, spending her days in the forest with her posse of animals. She is often pictured with a bow and arrow.

Summon the spirit of Artemis when you are in need of more power and strength. Call upon her when you need a guardian to protect you. She is also of service when you need to summon your strength for heading into battle, or even childbirth.

A Prayer for Artemis

Dear Artemis, please allow me to have more focus, determination, and drive. Allow my ambition to benefit my life and to better the planet. Please give me your wisdom and your tools so that I may accomplish my goals. Allow me to hone my animal-like instincts to strengthen my intuitive powers.

Sacred Objects for Artemis

Found items from nature, like leaves, sticks, rocks, and feathers; fire (like a candle or a fire you build in her honor in the fireplace); arrowheads; arrows; sandalwood or patchouli essential oil; butterflies; insect wings; bones; teeth; animal skins; pictures of beloved pets.

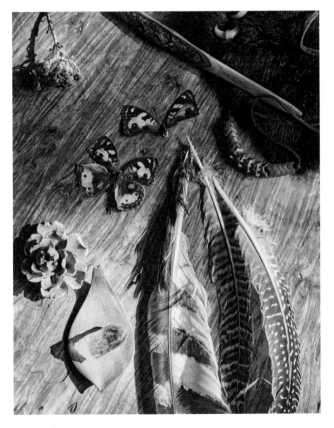

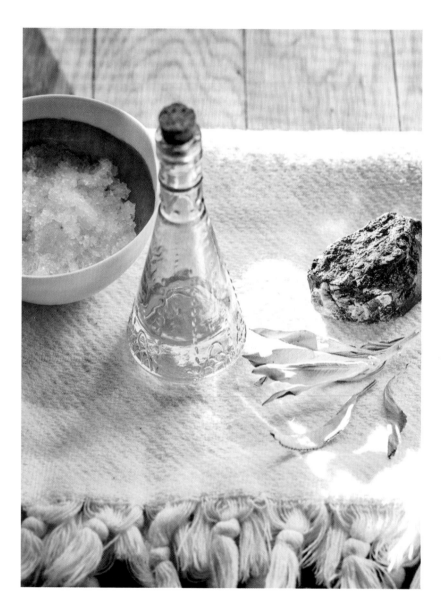

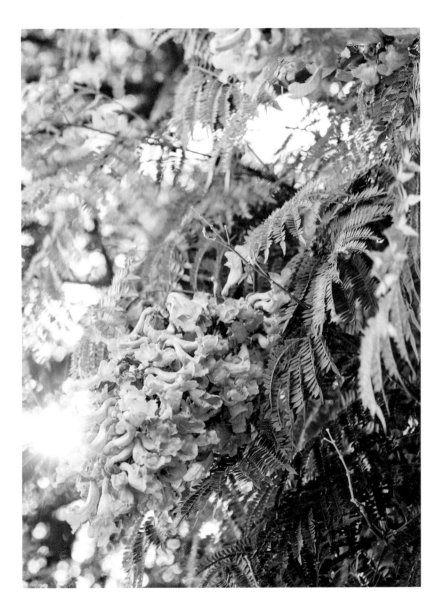

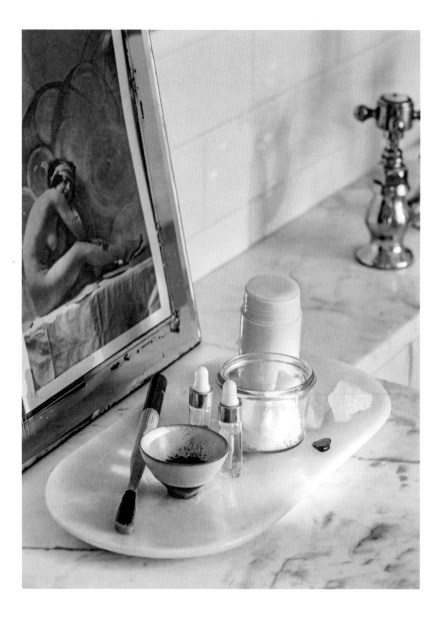

Deodorant

Around the age of twenty, I developed a lump beneath my armpit. There wasn't a ton of information about this at the time, but I began to do some research and became aware of the toxic implications of using traditional antiperspirants and deodorants made with aluminum. This was back in the early nineties when there wasn't a Whole Foods on every corner, and the internet wasn't what it is today, so I began to hunt for more "natural" choices at mom-and-pop health food stores. The only deodorants I could find were the crystal kind—which didn't work—so I began to make my own, one of my first forays into DIY products. Shortly after I stopped using traditional antiperspirants, the lump disappeared. This recipe is for a deodorant, not an antiperspirant. As inconvenient as it may be at times, you want to sweat! Sweating is an important part of your body's detoxification process.

⅓ cup coconut oil, at room temperature

2 tablespoons organic baking soda

⅓ cup arrowroot powder (easy to find at
   health food stores)

8 drops of rose essential oil

8 drops of sandalwood essential oil

Mason jar

Continued

Place the coconut oil in a small bowl and add the baking soda and arrowroot powder. Mash together with a wooden spoon until the mixture has the consistency of deodorant (white and chalky, yet not too crumbly). Add the essential oils. Transfer to the mason jar and use your fingers to rub it under your arms until it is absorbed. Wait to dress until after it has dried, to avoid smearing it on your clothes. Stored out of direct sunlight, it will keep for 6 to 9 months.

Toothpaste

I am wary of overexposure to fluoride. You will
be getting some naturally, as it is in most tap
water, so having fluoride in your toothpaste
is often redundant and could be harmful if
not monitored. Coconut oil is known to be an
antibacterial agent, and it helps fight tooth
decay. To increase the whitening effect, you can
add a drop of hydrogen peroxide to the paste.

3 tablespoons organic baking soda

3 tablespoons coconut oil

2 teaspoons glycerin

A few drops of stevia or 1 packet of xylitol (which also
    fights tooth decay)

20 drops of peppermint or cinnamon oil

Glass jar with lid

Mix the baking soda, coconut oil, glycerin, and stevia
or xylitol together in a bowl (it helps if the coconut
oil is a little warm), then add the peppermint or
cinnamon oil. Tightly close the lid and shake to mix.
Transfer to the glass jar. To use, sprinkle some of
the powder onto your toothbrush. Stored out of
direct sunlight, it will keep for 6 to 9 months.

Insect Repellent

Studies have shown that blends of lemon and eucalyptus oils can repel mosquitoes as effectively as toxic DEET. As always, this is something you should discuss with your physician, as there are many serious bug-borne illnesses.

½ cup water

¼ cup witch hazel

45 drops of eucalyptus oil

30 drops of lemon oil

10 drops of peppermint oil

6-ounce glass spray bottle

Combine the water and witch hazel with the eucalyptus, lemon, and peppermint oils in the spray bottle, and shake well before using. Apply often. Stored out of direct sunlight, it will keep for 6 to 9 months.

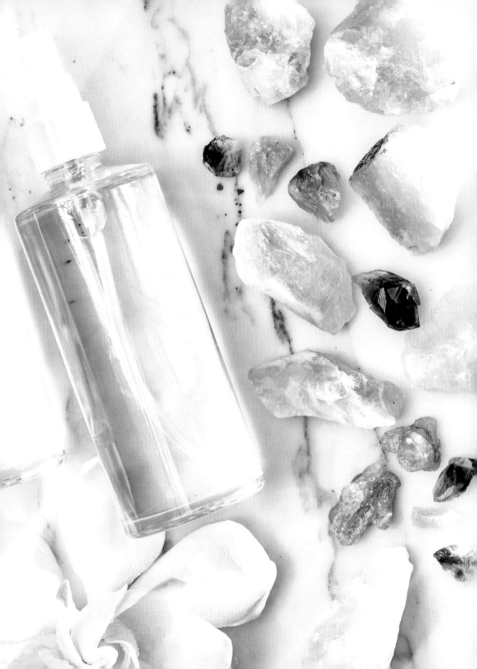

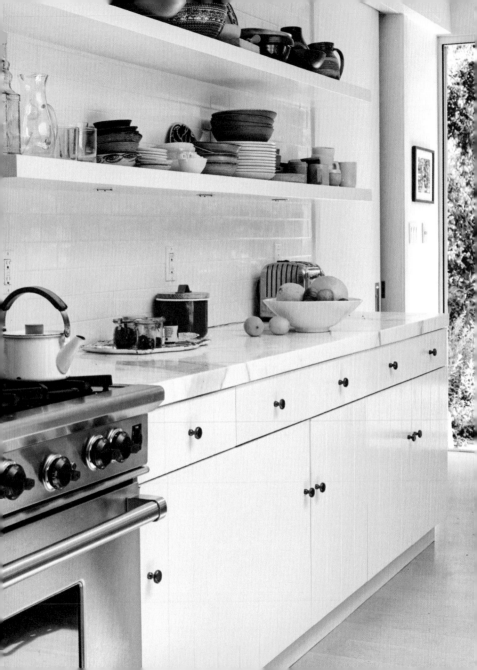

Cleaning with Essential Oils

Essential oils have helped me rid my home of
toxic cleaners. Note that in spite of their name,
essential oils are rarely oily, so don't worry
about using them in the following preparations.
They won't leave a greasy film behind.

Dishwashing Liquid

2 cups water

¼ cup soap flakes

¼ cup castile soap (I like Dr. Bronner's)

1 teaspoon glycerin

2 teaspoons washing soda (easy to find at hardware stores or superstores)

Essential oils of your choosing (see below)

Glass bottle with spout

For a Citrus Version

15 drops of grapefruit oil

15 drops of lemon oil

For an Evergreen Version

15 drops of cedar oil

15 drops of juniper oil

For a Floral Version

15 drops of geranium oil

15 drops of lavender oil

Bring the water to a low boil in a pot, then add the soap flakes and stir until they've dissolved. Remove from the heat to let cool, add the castile soap, glycerin, washing soda, and the essential oils of your choosing, and pour into the glass bottle. Shake well before each use. Stored out of direct sunlight, it will keep for up to 6 months.

Bleach Alternative

10 cups water
¼ cup lemon juice
1 cup hydrogen peroxide
10 drops of lemon oil

Water jug

Mix the water, lemon juice, hydrogen peroxide, and lemon oil in the water jug, and use 1 cup for each load of whites. Stored out of direct sunlight, it will keep for up to 6 months.

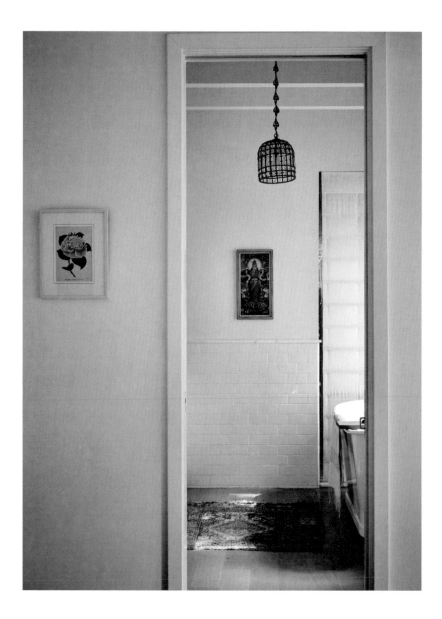

Surface & Floor Cleaner

½ cup white vinegar

½ gallon water

2 tablespoons organic baking soda

Essential oils of your choosing (see below)

Glass spray bottle (you can also use plastic, but
   I prefer glass to avoid exposure to phthalates
   and BPA) or metal bucket

For a Citrus Version

10 drops of grapefruit oil

10 drops of lemon oil

For an Evergreen Version

10 drops of cedar oil

10 drops of juniper oil

For a Floral Version

10 drops of geranium oil

10 drops of lavender oil

Mix the vinegar, water, and baking soda in the spray
bottle or bucket, and add the essential oils of your
choosing. To use, shake or stir well, then apply and
wipe or mop clean. Stored out of direct sunlight, it
will keep for up to 6 months.

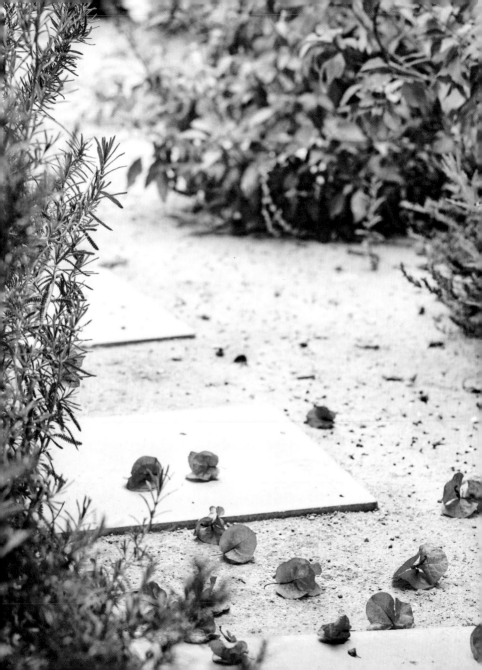

Essential Oils & Spiritual Practices

In some practices, essential oils are used to help correct any imbalances within the body and to invigorate us with renewed vitality. The following rituals—one Ayurvedic and one Kundalini—allow you to focus and tune in to what your body needs, and can trigger a profound shift into a more self-healing modality.

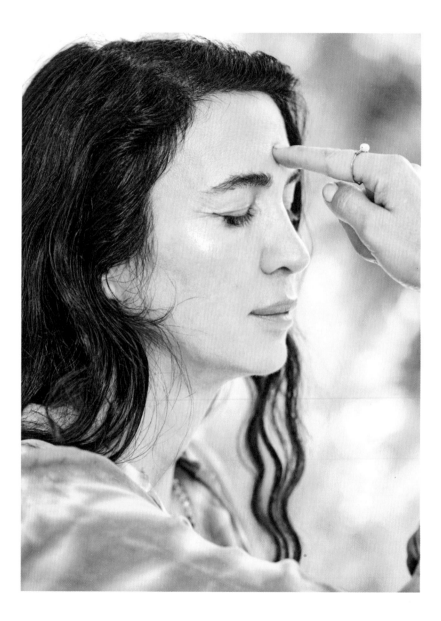

Anointing Your Doshas

Ayurvedic medicine is an ancient Indian healing practice that is all about connecting to ourselves and staying in harmony and balance with the natural world. Its core belief is that people are made up of three doshas, or life-giving forces: Vata, Pitta, and Kapha. Doshas are considered the inherent wisdom of the body and fuel the function of our bodies. Each dosha is made up of a combination of some of the five elements: air, water, earth, fire, and ether. According to Ayurveda, all health issues arise from an imbalance of the five elements. When the three doshas are perfectly aligned, you are considered healthy. Most of us have all of the doshas, but one of them is usually prominent. To identify the prominent one, you can take self-assessment quizzes on Ayurvedic websites such as Banyan Botanicals or the Chopra Center, or see an Ayurvedic practitioner. (You can find one through the National Ayurvedic Medical Association.) There is also an abundance of information about Ayurveda in books and online (see Resources).

Anointing yourself with essential oils is an empowering way to shift your energy, take control of your vision for what you want in your life, and help to balance your doshas. To do this, I like to take a few drops of the appropriate oil on my finger, and start at the top of my head. I work down from the crown of my head, to my third eye, then to my heart, then to right below my belly button, to my pubic bone, and finally to the soles of my feet. As I do so, I also imagine that I am activating my chakras and flooding them with pure, positive light.

The Doshas

Vata

Vata is a combination of air and ether. This dosha promotes mobility, activity, and breath. When Vata is balanced, we can easily evoke joy, happiness, and lightness of being. When it's out of balance, we might feel fearful, anxious, and nervous. A person dominant in Vata will typically be underweight, with poor circulation and rough or dry skin. He or she will walk quickly, have a quick mind, and crave sweet and sour foods, like chocolate and lemons.

Pitta

Pitta is a combination of fire and water. This dosha controls our digestion, metabolism, and energy production. When Pitta is balanced, we are moving, thinking, and understanding things really quickly. When it's out of balance, we might experience

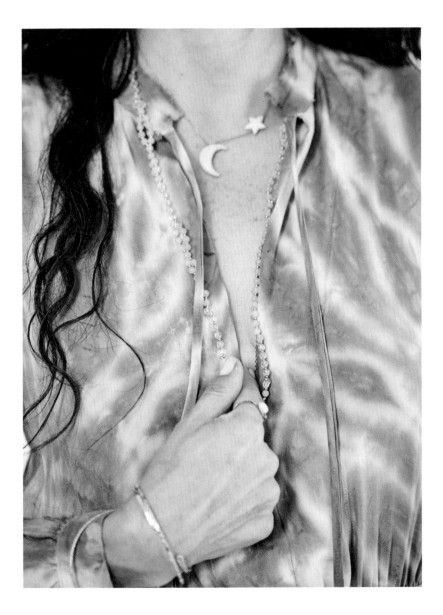

frustration, anger, and argumentative behavior. A person dominant in Pitta will typically be of medium build, with a warm body temperature and oily skin. He or she will be a night owl, with intense cravings for greasy foods like pizza and French fries, and spicy foods like hot sauce.

Kapha

Kapha is a combination of earth and water. This dosha is the energetic force behind the body's structure, what holds cells together and forms bone, muscle, fat, and sinew. With Kapha in balance, we feel harmonious, full of love, and calm. When it's out of balance, we'll often feel stubborn and resistant to change. A person dominant in Kapha might have a larger frame and be a bit heavier. He or she might feel sluggish and have a strong craving for sweets.

TO CALM VATA

Clary Sage · Geranium ·
Jasmine · Musk · Rose ·
Sandalwood

TO COOL PITTA

Gardenia · Jasmine · Melissa ·
Mint · Rose

TO STIMULATE KAPHA

Cedar · Cinnamon · Myrrh ·
Patchouli · Pine · Sage

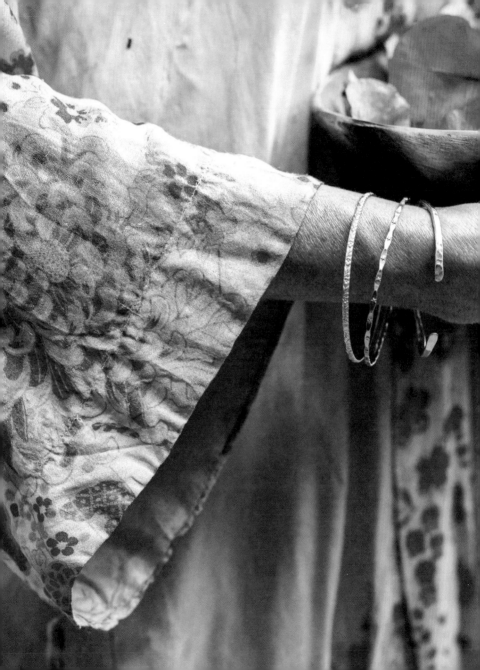

Activating Your Chakras with Essential Oils

Almost fifteen years ago, I was on Kauai and received a body treatment from an angelic woman who told me that my chakras seemed shut down. I was physically, spiritually, and emotionally depleted, struggling to just make it through each day. I was depressed, and the autoimmune issues I had struggled with throughout my life were flaring up. At the time, I didn't really understand what chakras were, but I knew that something wasn't working, and the words of this woman unlocked a window in my mind.

When I finally started my wellness journey, I found myself returning again and again to my chakras, intent on getting them open and spinning. After years of Kundalini practice, I am well attuned to the powers of the seven chakras.

Each one has a front and a back, the front connecting to your emotions and the back connecting to your will. Each also corresponds to a different part of your physical body. Problems with the chakras in the subtle body, which is the energy field that extends beyond your physical body, will eventually lead to health issues and injury. The chakras' coordinates are represented as a rainbow: red is earth, and the colors get cooler as you move up into the atmosphere.

Meditating on certain chakras can help put them into motion, but you can also activate them by massaging the corresponding parts on your body with essential oils. Since the chakras are yearning to be opened and flowing, essential oils are a powerful tool to help this along. If you're feeling ungrounded, reach for an earthy, wood-based essential oil. Just by placing a few drops on your feet, you'll feel a deeper connection to the earth. Or try placing rose essential oil on your heart chakra, and feel your whole body soften. This is something you can experiment with; feel the subtle changes occurring with each use. Our chakras will absorb everything, so using pure essential oils is a must.

There are seven chakras.

First Chakra

This chakra, also known as the root chakra, is located just below your stomach in the sacral area around the groin and is about feeling grounded and connected to the earth. It is the chakra of your most basic needs, what you must have in your life before you can begin to ascend to higher levels. When the first chakra is spinning, you feel safe, confident, and supported.

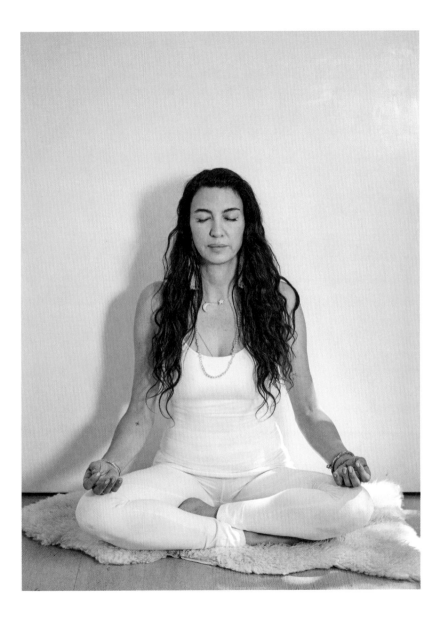

ASSOCIATIONS

Color: Red

Corresponding glands: Ovaries, testes

Symptoms of a stuck first chakra: Feeling
ungrounded, disconnected

Essential oils: Cedarwood, myrrh, patchouli

Second Chakra

This is the chakra of creativity. It is located in your
lower belly and allows you to create something
out of nothing, giving birth to everything from
children to artistic projects. When the second
chakra is spinning, you feel creative and at ease.

ASSOCIATIONS

Color: Orange

Corresponding glands: Adrenal

Symptoms of a stuck second chakra: Feeling trapped

Essential oils: Bergamot, clary sage, jasmine, ylang-
ylang

Third Chakra

This is your energy chakra and the source of
your personal power. It is what enables you to
manifest your desires and is located in the center

of your belly. When the third chakra is spinning, you feel energetic and driven, equipped with the will and confidence to go after what you want.

ASSOCIATIONS

Color: Yellow

Corresponding gland: Pancreas

Symptoms of a stuck third chakra: Feeling tired, frustrated, insecure

Essential oils: Cinnamon, geranium, ginger, juniper, lemon, rosemary, sandalwood

Fourth Chakra

This is your heart chakra. It is the seat of love, forgiveness, trust, and compassion and is located in the center of your chest. When the fourth chakra is spinning, you feel deep love for and connection with those around you. You are able to freely give and receive love in all its many forms.

ASSOCIATIONS

Color: Green

Corresponding gland: Thymus

Symptoms of a stuck fourth chakra: Feeling lonely, alienated, unable to forgive or accept forgiveness

Essential oils: Cypress, Melissa, rose, ylang-ylang

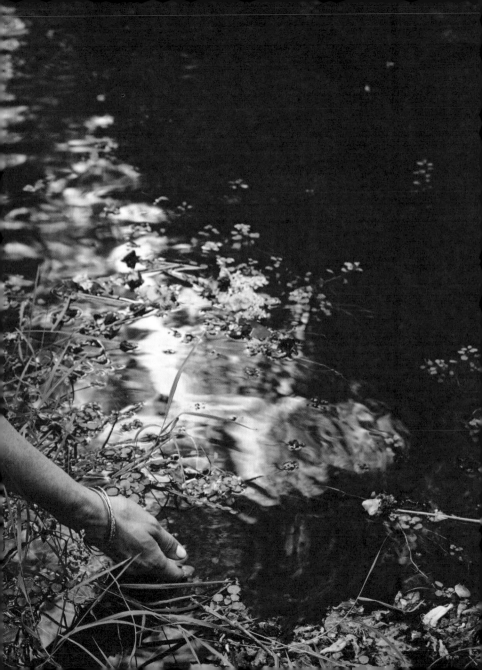

Fifth Chakra

This is the throat chakra and rules your ability to express yourself. It governs communication, speaking, and writing. When this chakra is spinning, you feel that your voice is being heard and that you are empowered to speak your truth and ask for what you want.

ASSOCIATIONS
Color: Blue
Corresponding gland: Thyroid
Symptoms of a stuck fifth chakra: Feeling anxious about others' opinions of you, unable to speak up
Essential oils: Basil, chamomile, cypress, palmarosa, peppermint

Sixth Chakra

This is the intuition chakra. Located in the center of your forehead, it governs your sixth sense and psychic abilities. The sixth chakra is your inner voice that guides you to trust your instincts. When it is balanced, you are able to tap in to your inner guidance without fear.

ASSOCIATIONS
Color: Lavender
Corresponding gland: Pituitary

Symptoms of a stuck sixth chakra: Feeling doubtful, indecisive, unsure of what you want

Essential oils: Bay, cedarwood, clary sage, frankincense, helichrysum, sandalwood

Seventh Chakra

This is the crown chakra. Imagine it as a thousand-petaled lotus flower blooming at the top of your head. When all of your other chakras are spinning, the lotus begins to bloom. You connect to the source of all being and recognize your own divinity.

ASSOCIATIONS

Color: Violet

Corresponding gland: Pineal

Symptoms of a stuck seventh chakra: Feeling materialistic and not living consciously

Essential oils: Frankincense, lavender, myrrh, sandalwood

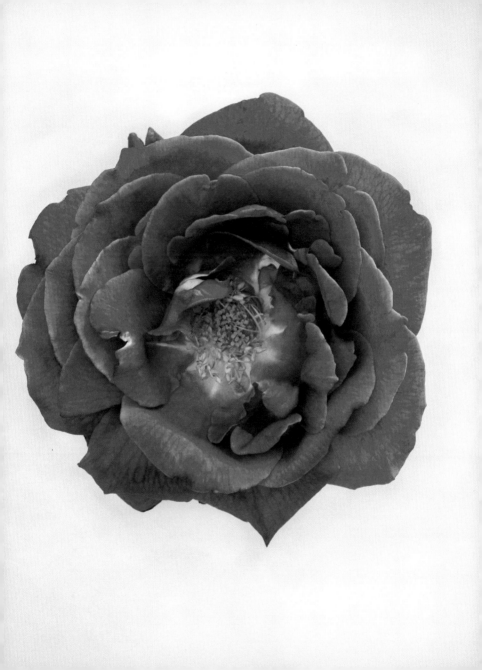

When we treat our body, our vessel, with intention, we are honoring not just ourselves but the essence of femininity that has coursed through us since the beginning of time.

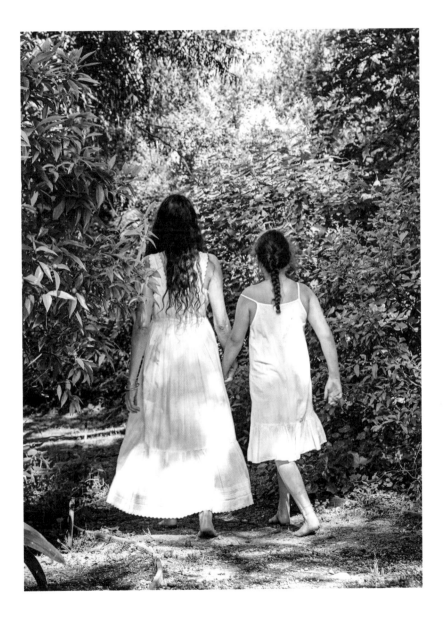

FURTHER READING

In addition to in my blog, *The Local Rose*, my writing has appeared on the following websites.

TheChalkboardMag.com
Goop.com
MindBodyGreen.com

These are a few books I recommend.

The Complete Book of Essential Oils and Aromatherapy, by Valerie Ann Worwood

The Goddess Pages: A Divine Guide to Finding Love and Happiness, by Laurie Sue Brockway

Love Is in the Earth: A Kaleidoscope of Crystals, by Melody

RESOURCES

Learn more about holistic living and my products on TheLocalRose.com. In addition, these are the websites I frequently visit to shop for ingredients and seek out new insights and information.

Ayurveda
BanyanBotanicals.com
Chopra.com
SuryaSpa.com

To find an Ayurvedic practitioner
in your area:
AyurvedaNAMA.org

Crystals
CrystalsMtShasta.com

Essential Oils
EdensGarden.com
LivingLibations.com

Spices & Ingredients
BanyanBotanicals.com
DualSpices.com

Copyright © 2018, 2019 by Shiva Rose
Photographs copyright © 2018 by Ngoc Minh Ngo
Illustrations copyright © 2018 by Spiros Halaris

All rights reserved. No portion of this book may be reproduced—
mechanically, electronically, or by any other means, including
photocopying—without written permission of the publisher.

Library of Congress Cataloging-in-Publication Data

Names: Rose, Shiva, author.
Title: Whole beauty : essential oils : homemade recipes for clean
    beauty and household care / Shiva Rose.
Description: New York : Artisan, a division of
    Workman Publishing Co., Inc. [2019]
Identifiers: LCCN 2018030082 | ISBN 9781579659042
    (hardcover : alk. paper)
Subjects: LCSH: Essences and essential oils.
Classification: LCC TP958 .R775 2019 | DDC 661/.806—dc23 LC
    record available at https://lccn.loc.gov/2018030082

33614080909186

Artisan books are available at special discounts when purchased in
bulk for premiums and sales promotions as well as for fund-raising or
educational use. Special editions or book excerpts also can be created
to specification. For details, contact the Special Sales Director at the
address below, or send an e-mail to specialmarkets@workman.com.

For speaking engagements, contact speakersbureau@workman.com.

Published by Artisan
A division of Workman Publishing Co., Inc.
225 Varick Street
New York, NY 10014-4381
artisanbooks.com

Artisan is a registered trademark of Workman Publishing Co., Inc.

This book has been adapted from *Whole Beauty* (Artisan, 2018).

Design adapted from CHD

Published simultaneously in Canada by Thomas Allen & Son, Limited `

Printed in China
First printing, February 2019

10 9 8 7 6 5 4 3 2 1